Related Kaplan Books

Get Into Medical School: A Strategic Approach

MCAT Biological Sciences Flashcards

MCAT Comprehensive Review with CD-ROM

MCAT Practice Tests

MCAT 45

KAPLAN

MCAT®

Physical Sciences Flashcards

By the Staff of Kaplan, Inc.

Simon & Schuster

NEW YORK · LONDON · SYDNEY · TORONTO

Kaplan Publishing
Published by Simon & Schuster
1230 Avenue of the Americas
New York, NY 10020

Contributing Editor: Albert Chen
Editorial Director: Jennifer Farthing
Editor: Larissa Shmailo
Production Manager: Michael Shevlin
Content Manager: Vanessa Torrado-Caputo
Cover Design: Cheung Tai
Interior Page Layout: Dave Chipps

June 2005

10 9 8 7 6 5 4 3 2
Manufactured in the United States of America
Published simultaneously in Canada

ISBN 0-7432-7141-6

How to Use This Book

Kaplan's *MCAT® Physical Sciences Flashcards* is perfectly designed to help you learn 350 basic MCAT physical sciences concepts in a quick, easy, and fun way. Simply read the MCAT category (Physics or General Chemistry) and the item name on the front of the flashcard; then flip to the back to see its definition and subcategory.

The following categories and subcategories have been included in the book.

General Chemistry

- Atomic Structure
- The Periodic Table
- Bonding
- Compounds and Stoichiometry
- Kinetics and Equilibrium
- Thermochemistry
- The Gas Phase
- Phase and Phase Changes
- Solutions
- Acids and Bases
- Redox Reactions and Electrochemistry

Physics

Units and Kinematics
Newtonian Mechanics
Work, Energy, and Momentum
Thermodynamics
Fluids and Solids
Electrostatics
Magnetism
DC and AC Circuits
Periodic Motions, Waves, and Sound
Light and Optics
Atomic Phenomena
Nuclear Phenomena

Once you've mastered a particular item, clip or fold back the corner of the flashcard so that you can zip right by it on your next pass through the book. This Flashcard book is packed with information—remember to flip the book over and flip through the other half!

Looking for still more MCAT® exam prep? Be sure to pick up a copy of Kaplan's comprehensive *MCAT® Comprehensive Review with CD-ROM*, complete with a full-length practice test.

Good luck!

General Chemistry

ATOM

Nuclear Phenomena

An anti-electron, denoted β+ or e+, emitted in a nuclear reaction.

Atomic Structure

The basic building block of all matter in the universe. An atom is made up of three main components: protons, neutrons, and electrons.

POSITRON

Physics

General Chemistry

ATOMIC ABSORPTION SPECTRUM

Nuclear Phenomena

The difference between an atom's atomic mass and the sum of its protons and neutrons.

Atomic Structure

The spectrum of certain absorbed wavelengths of light corresponding to an atom's spectrum of emitted frequencies of light.

MASS DEFECT

Physics

ATOMIC EMISSION SPECTRA

Nuclear Phenomena

The amount of time it takes for one-half of a radioactive sample to decay, given by the equation $T_{1/2} = \ln 2/\lambda$, where λ is a decay constant.

Atomic Structure

The discontinuous line spectra of light produced when excited atoms return to their ground state and emit photons of a certain frequency.

HALF-LIFE

Physics

General Chemistry

ATOMIC MASS UNIT

Nuclear Phenomena

The atomic emission of high energy photons, also known as γ-particles.

Atomic Structure

The unit of mass equal to 1/12 the mass (in grams) of a carbon-12 atom; 1 amu is approximately equal to the mass of a proton.

GAMMA DECAY

Physics

General Chemistry

ATOMIC NUMBER

Nuclear Phenomena

The nuclear reaction in which two or more small nuclei combine to form a larger nucleus.

Atomic Structure

The number of protons in an element, often denoted by the letter "Z."

FUSION

Physics

General Chemistry

ATOMIC WEIGHT

Nuclear Phenomena

The nuclear reaction in which a large nucleus splits up into smaller nuclei.

Atomic Structure

The average mass, measured in amu, of all the isotopes of a given element as they occur naturally.

FISSION

Physics

General Chemistry

AUFBAU PRINCIPLE

Nuclear Phenomena

A decrease in the amount of substance N given by the equation: $N = N_0 \times e^{-\lambda t}$.

Atomic Structure

Electrons fill an atom in order of increasing energy level.

EXPONENTIAL DECAY

Physics

AZIMUTHAL QUANTUM NUMBER

Nuclear Phenomena

A radioactive process in which a nucleus captures an inner-shell electron that combines with a proton to form a neutron. As a result, the atomic number decreases by 1, but the atomic mass remains the same.

Atomic Structure

The second quantum number. Designated by the letter *l*, it means "angular momentum" and refers to the subshells within each principle quantum energy level. *l* can take on the value of an integer in the 0 to $n - 1$ range.

ELECTRON CAPTURE

Physics

BALMER SERIES

Nuclear Phenomena

The energy that holds the protons and neutrons together in the nucleus, defined by the equation $E = mc^2$, where m is the mass defect and c is the speed of light in a vacuum.

Atomic Structure

A set of spectral lines that appear in the visible light region when a hydrogen atom undergoes a transition from energy levels $n > 2$ to $n = 2$.

BINDING ENERGY

Physics

THE BOHR MODEL

Nuclear Phenomena

Nuclear reaction in which a β-particle (e^-) is emitted.

Atomic Structure

A model of the atom postulating that electrons are located in discrete circular orbits about the nucleus. In this model, the electrostatic force between the positive nucleus and negative electron acts as the centripetal force keeping the electron in orbit.

BETA DECAY

Physics

Nuclear Phenomena

Nuclear reaction in which an α-particle ($_2^4He$) is emitted.

DIAMAGNETIC

General Chemistry

Atomic Structure

An atom or a substance that contains no unpaired electrons and is consequently repelled by a magnet.

Physics

ALPHA DECAY

ELECTRON

Atomic Phenomena

The minimum amount of photon energy required to emit an electron from a certain metal. This quantity, denoted by W, is used to calculate the residual kinetic energy of an electron emitted by a metal, given by: $KE = hf - W$, where hf is the energy of a photon.

Atomic Structure

A subatomic particle that orbits the nucleus and has a charge of −1. The electron has a negligible mass and is often denoted by the symbol e^-.

WORK FUNCTION

Physics

General Chemistry

ELECTRON CONFIGURATION

Atomic Phenomena

The phenomenon observed when light of a certain frequency is incident on a sheet of metal and causes it to emit an electron.

Atomic Structure

The patterned order by which electrons fill subshells and energy levels in an atom. The first number designates the principle quantum number (n), the letter—s, p, d, f, g—specifies the subshell (l), and the superscript indicates the number of electrons in that subshell.

PHOTOELECTRIC EFFECT

Physics

HEISENBERG UNCERTAINTY PRINCIPLE

Atomic Phenomena

The phenomenon observed when an atom is excited by UV light and the electrons return to the ground state in two or more steps, emitting photons of lower frequency (often in the visible light spectrum) at each step.

Atomic Structure

The quantum mechanical idea that we cannot measure the exact momentum and position of an orbiting electron simultaneously. That is, the more accurately we measure an electron's momentum, the less we know about its exact position.

FLUORESCENCE

Physics

General Chemistry

HUND'S RULE

Light and Optics

An image produced at a point where light does not actually pass or converge. For mirrors this would be on the opposite site of the object; for lenses it would be on the same side as the object.

Atomic Structure

Electrons will first fill equal-energy orbitals of a subshell unpaired and with parallel spins before being coupled with other electrons of opposite spins in the same orbital. This method of maximizing the number of half-filled orbitals allows for the most stable distribution of electrons within a subshell.

VIRTUAL IMAGE

Physics

General Chemistry

ISOELECTRONIC

Light and Optics

The condition in which the θ_1 of light traveling from a medium with a high n to a medium with a low n is greater than the critical angle θ_c, resulting in all of the light being reflected and none of it being refracted.

Atomic Structure

Two different elements that share the same electronic configuration. Example: K+ and Ar.

TOTAL INTERNAL REFLECTION

Physics

General Chemistry

ISOTOPES

Light and Optics

A curved mirror that is essentially a small, cut-out portion of a sphere mirror, having a center of curvature C and radius of curvature r.

Atomic Structure

Atoms sharing the same atomic number (Z) but a different number of neutrons.

SPHERICAL MIRROR

Physics

LYMAN SERIES

Light and Optics

The speed of electromagnetic waves traveling through a vacuum, given by the equation $c = \lambda f$, where c is a constant, is equal to 3.00×10^8 m/s.

Atomic Structure

A set of spectral lines that appear in the UV region when a hydrogen atom undergoes a transition from energy levels $n > 1$ to $n = 1$.

SPEED OF LIGHT

Physics

General Chemistry

MAGNETIC QUANTUM NUMBER

Light and Optics

Equation describing the angle of refraction for a light ray passing from one medium to another, given by $n_1\sin\theta_1 = n_2\sin\theta_2$, where n is the index of refraction.

Atomic Structure

The third quantum number. Designated by m_l, it describes a particular orbital within a subshell where an electron is very likely to be found. The possible values for m_l are integers in the $-l$ to l range, including 0.

SNELL'S LAW

Physics

General Chemistry

MASS NUMBER

Light and Optics

An image produced at a point where the light rays actually converge or pass through. For mirrors this would be on the side of the object; for lenses it would be on the opposite side of the object.

Atomic Structure

Sum of the protons and neutrons in an element, often denoted by the letter "A."

REAL IMAGE

Physics

General Chemistry

NEUTRON

Light and Optics

Light that has been passed through a polarizing filter, only allowing the transmission of waves containing electric field vectors parallel to the lines of the filter.

Atomic Structure

A subatomic particle with zero electric charge that is slightly heavier than a proton.

PLANE-POLARIZED LIGHT

Physics

General Chemistry

NUCLEUS

Light and Optics

A mirror in which incident light rays remain parallel after reflection, always producing a virtual image that appears to be the same distance behind the mirror as the object is in front of the mirror.

Atomic Structure

The dense, positively charged center of an atom containing its protons and neutrons.

PLANE MIRROR

Physics

General Chemistry

ORBITAL

Light and Optics

A dimensionless value denoted by m given by the equation: $m = -i/o$, where i is image height and o is object height. A negative m denotes an inverted image whereas a positive m denotes an upright image.

Atomic Structure

A three-dimensional region about the nucleus where a rapidly orbiting electron is likely to be found. Each orbital has a unique assignment of values for the *n*, *l*, and m_l quantum numbers.

MAGNIFICATION

Physics

General Chemistry

PARAMAGNETIC

Light and Optics

Law stating that when light waves strike a medium the angle of incidence θ_i is equal to the angle of reflection θ_r.

Atomic Structure

An atom or a substance that contains unpaired electrons and is consequently attracted by a magnet.

LAW OF REFLECTION

Physics

General Chemistry

PASCHEN SERIES

Light and Optics

When superimposed light waves are in phase, their amplitudes add (constructive interference) and the appearance is brighter. When superimposed light waves are out of phase, their amplitudes subtract (destructive interference) and the appearance is darker.

Atomic Structure

A set of spectral lines resulting when a hydrogen atom undergoes a transition from energy levels $n \geq 4$ to $n = 3$.

INTERFERENCE

Physics

General Chemistry

PAULI EXCLUSION PRINCIPLE

Light and Optics

Ratio of the speed of light in a vacuum to the speed of light though a medium, given by: $n = c/v$; factor by which the c is reduced as light travels from a vacuum into another medium.

Atomic Structure

No two electrons in an atom can have the same set of four quantum number values.

INDEX OF REFRACTION

Physics

General Chemistry

PFUND SERIES

Light and Optics

The distance between the focal point and the mirror or lens. For spherical mirrors the focal length is equal to one-half the radius of curvature.

Atomic Structure

A set of spectral lines resulting when a hydrogen atom undergoes a transition from energy levels $n > 5$ to $n = 5$.

FOCAL LENGTH

Physics

Light and Optics

When a magnetic field is changing it causes a change in an electric field and visa versa, resulting in the propagation of a transverse wave containing a magnetic and electric field that are perpendicular to each other.

PHOTON

General Chemistry

Atomic Structure

A unit of energy in the form of light equal to *hf*, where *h* is Planck's constant and *f* is the frequency of radiation.

ELECTROMAGNETIC WAVES

Physics

General Chemistry

PRINCIPLE QUANTUM NUMBER

Light and Optics

The full range of frequencies and wavelengths for electromagnetic waves broken down into the following regions (in descending order of λ): radio, infrared, visible light, ultraviolet, x-ray, and gamma ray.

Atomic Structure

The first quantum number. Designated by the letter *n*, it takes on any positive integer value and describes an electron's energy level. An electron with a higher *n* value is at a higher energy state.

ELECTROMAGNETIC SPECTRUM

Physics

General Chemistry

PROTON

Light and Optics

A convex mirror with a negative focal length. Diverging mirrors always produce virtual images.

Atomic Structure

A subatomic particle with a charge of +1 and mass of 1.0073 amu.

DIVERGING MIRROR

Physics

General Chemistry

QUANTUM MECHANICS

A lens with a thin center that diverges light after refraction and always forms a virtual image.

Light and Optics

Atomic Structure

Study of physics at the atomic level where energy is quantized in discrete, rather than continuous, levels.

DIVERGING LENS

Physics

Light and Optics

The phenomenon observed when white light is incident on the face of a prism and emerges on the opposite side with all its wavelengths split apart. This occurs because λ is related to the index of refraction by the relationship: $n = c/f\lambda$. Therefore, a small λ has a large n and, in turn, a small angle of refraction θ_2).

QUANTUM NUMBERS

General Chemistry

Atomic Structure

A set of four numbers used to describe an electron's energy state (position and energy).

Physics

DISPERSION

SPIN QUANTUM NUMBER

The spreading-out effect of light when it passes through a small slit opening.

Atomic Structure

The fourth quantum number. Designated by m_s, it specifies an electron's intrinsic spin value or angular momentum in an orbital. Since there can be no more than two electrons per orbital, the value of m_s can only be +1/2 or –1/2.

DIFFRACTION

Physics

General Chemistry

VALENCE ELECTRONS

Light and Optics

A concave mirror with a positive focal length.

Atomic Structure

The electrons occupying the outermost electron shell of an atom that participate in chemical bonds. Atoms with the same number of valence electrons usually have similar properties.

Physics

CONVERGING MIRROR

General Chemistry

ALKALI METALS

Light and Optics

A lens with a thick center that converges light rays at a point where the image is formed.

The Periodic Table

The highly reactive elements found in Group IA of the Periodic Table, except hydrogen.

CONVERGING LENS

Physics

General Chemistry

ALKALINE EARTHS

Periodic Motions, Waves, and Sound

The speed of a wave, which is related to the frequency and wavelength by the equation $v = f\lambda$.

The Periodic Table

Elements found in Group IIA of the Periodic Table.

WAVE SPEED

Physics

ATOMIC RADIUS

Periodic Motions, Waves, and Sound

A quantity equal to the distance between any two equivalent consecutive points along a wave, such as two consecutive crest peaks; λ.

The Periodic Table

The distance measured either between the nucleus and outermost electron of an atom or by the separation of the two nuclei in a diatomic element. Decreases from left to right and bottom to top on the periodic table.

WAVELENGTH

Physics

General Chemistry

EFFECTIVE NUCLEAR CHARGE

Periodic Motions, Waves, and Sound

Type of wave, such as light, whose oscillation is perpendicular to its direction of motion.

The Periodic Table

The resulting positive nuclear charge an outer electron senses after accounting for the shielding effect of inner core electrons. Abbreviated Z_{eff}. Increases from left to right and bottom to top on the periodic table.

TRANSVERSE WAVE

Physics

General Chemistry

ELECTRON AFFINITY

Periodic Motions, Waves, and Sound

A measure of a spring's stiffness, denoted by k.

The Periodic Table

The energy released when an atom or ion in the gaseous state gains an electron. Increases from left to right and bottom to top on the periodic table.

SPRING CONSTANT

Physics

General Chemistry

ELECTRONEGATIVITY

Periodic Motions, Waves, and Sound

A quantity measured in decibels (dB) and denoted by β, given by the equation: $\beta = 10 \log I/I_0$ where I_0 is a reference intensity of 10^{-12} W/m^2.

The Periodic Table

A measure of an atom's ability to pull electron density toward itself when involved in a chemical bond. Increases from left to right and bottom to top on the periodic table.

SOUND LEVEL

Physics

General Chemistry

FREE RADICAL

Periodic Motions, Waves, and Sound

The motion of an object oscillating back and forth about some equilibrium point when it is subject to an elastic linear restoring force.

The Periodic Table

An atom or molecule that has an unpaired electron in its outermost shell.

SIMPLE HARMONIC MOTION

Physics

General Chemistry

HALOGENS

Periodic Motions, Waves, and Sound

If a standing wave undergoes a forced oscillation due to an external periodic force that has a frequency equal to the natural frequency of the oscillating system, the amplitude will reach a maximum.

The Periodic Table

Elements found in Group VIIA of the Periodic Table.

RESONANCE

Physics

General Chemistry

IONIZATION ENERGY

Periodic Motions, Waves, and Sound

The angle by which the sine curve of one wave leads or lags the sine curve of another wave.

The Periodic Table

The amount of energy required to remove an electron from orbit about a gaseous atom into free space. Increases from left to right and bottom to top on the Periodic Table.

PHASE DIFFERENCE

Physics

General Chemistry

METALLOIDS

Periodic Motions, Waves, and Sound

Number of seconds it takes to complete one cycle, denoted by T; the inverse value of frequency.

The Periodic Table

B, Si, Ge, As, Sb, Te, and Po are called metalloids and have properties that are in between those of metals and nonmetals.

PERIOD

Physics

General Chemistry

METALS

Periodic Motions, Waves, and Sound

The point of zero displacement in a standing wave.

The Periodic Table

Elements that are characteristically electropositive, malleable, and ductile. These elements tend to be found the left side of the Periodic Table, lustrous, and have relatively low ionization energies and electron affinities.

NODE

Physics

General Chemistry

NOBLE GAS

Periodic Motions, Waves, and Sound

Type of wave, such as sound, whose oscillation is along the direction of its motion.

The Periodic Table

Inert elements naturally existing in a gaseous state that comprise Group VIII of the Periodic Table.

Physics

LONGITUDINAL WAVE

General Chemistry

NONMETALS

Periodic Motions, Waves, and Sound

The power transmitted per unit area, given by the equation $P = IA$, where I is intensity, A is area, and P is power.

The Periodic Table

Elements that have characteristically high electronegativity, ionization energy, and electron affinity. These elements tend to be found on the right side of the Periodic Table and are poor conductors of electricity.

General Chemistry

TRANSITION ELEMENTS

Periodic Motions, Waves, and Sound

The equation describing the restoring force of a mass-spring system, given by $F = -k\,x$, where x is the displacement from the equilibrium position.

The Periodic Table

The elements found in the B Groups of the Periodic Table. These elements contain partially filled d subshells.

HOOK'S LAW

Physics

General Chemistry

BOND ENERGY

Periodic Motions, Waves, and Sound

All the possible frequencies that a standing wave can support.

Bonding

The energy required to break one mole of a chemical bond; bond enthalpy.

HARMONIC SERIES

Physics

Periodic Motions, Waves, and Sound

The lowest frequency that a standing wave can support, given by the equation $f = nv/2L$ for strings fixed at both ends and pipes open at both ends and $f = nv/4L$ for pipes closed at one end, where $n = 1$; first harmonic.

COVALENT BOND

General Chemistry

Bonding

A chemical bond formed when atoms share bonding electron pairs.

FUNDAMENTAL FREQUENCY

Physics

General Chemistry

DIPOLE–DIPOLE INTERACTIONS

Periodic Motions, Waves, and Sound

Number of cycles per second measured in SI units of Hz, where 1 Hz = 1 cycle/second.

Bonding

Type of intermolecular force in which opposite poles of neighboring dipole molecules are drawn together.

FREQUENCY

Physics

Periodic Motions, Waves, and Sound

When a source emitting a sound and a detector receiving the sound move relative to each other, the virtual frequency fv' detected is less than or greater than the actual frequency emitted f, depending on whether the source and detector move toward or away from each other.

$f' = f\,(V \pm V_D)/(V \pm V_S)$.

DIPOLE MOMENT

General Chemistry

Bonding

The product of the amount of partial charge at either end of a molecule's dipole multiplied by the distance between them, given by the equation $p = qd$ where p is the dipole moment, q is the partial charge, and d is the distance separating the dipole.

DOPPLER EFFECT

Physics

DISPERSION FORCES

Periodic Motions, Waves, and Sound

When two overlapping waves are out of phase they subtract and can cancel each other out if they have the same amplitude and are 180 degrees out of phase.

Bonding

A weak intermolecular force prevalent in nonpolar covalent molecules caused by transient dipole-induced dipole attractions; a.k.a. London Forces.

DESTRUCTIVE INTERFERENCE

Physics

General Chemistry

FORMAL CHARGE

When two overlapping waves are in phase their amplitudes add together.

Periodic Motions, Waves, and Sound

Bonding

The charge assigned to an atom in a molecule or polyatomic ion calculated by the formula: # valence e^- – # 1/2 bonding e^- – # nonbonding e^-. Molecules containing atoms with lower formal charges tend to be more stable than those with higher formal charges.

Physics

CONSTRUCTIVE INTERFERENCE

Periodic Motions, Waves, and Sound

A periodic frequency resulting from the superposition of two waves that have slightly different frequencies, given by $f_{beat} = |f_1 - f_2|$.

HYDROGEN BONDING

General Chemistry

Bonding

Very strong intermolecular force where a hydrogen covalently bound to either a N, O, or F is attracted to another N, O, or F.

General Chemistry

INTERMOLECULAR FORCES

Periodic Motions, Waves, and Sound

The point of maximum displacement in a standing wave.

Bonding

The attractive and repulsive forces between neighboring molecules.

ANTI-NODE

Physics

General Chemistry

IONIC BOND

Periodic Motions, Waves, and Sound

A quantity denoted by ω that is equal to $\sqrt{k/m}$.

Bonding

A type of chemical bond in which there is a complete transfer of valence electrons to form positive and negative ions that are subsequently bound by electrostatic forces; strong attractions holding ions together in an ionic compound.

ANGULAR FREQUENCY

Physics

General Chemistry

LEWIS STRUCTURE

The point of maximum displacement from the equilibrium position.

Periodic Motions, Waves, and Sound

Bonding

A method using lines and dots to represent valence electrons and shared pairs of electrons of atoms, ions, or molecules.

AMPLITUDE

Physics

MOLECULAR ORBITAL

DC and AC Circuits

$V_{max}/\sqrt{2}$; The average voltage in an AC circuit, where the voltage alternates in a sinusoidal pattern.

Bonding

The region in a molecule where atomic orbitals overlap, resulting in either a stable low-energy bonding orbital or an unstable high-energy antibonding orbital.

RMS VOLTAGE

Physics

General Chemistry

NONPOLAR COVALENT BOND

DC and AC Circuits

$I_{max}/\sqrt{2}$: A quantity used to calculate the average power dissipated in an AC Circuit. This equation must be used because the average current, when calculated by conventional means, equals zero as a result of the periodic nature of that current.

Bonding

A type of covalent bond between atoms with the same electronegativities resulting in an even distribution of electron density along the bond.

RMS CURRENT

Physics

General Chemistry

OCTET RULE

DC and AC Circuits

Intrinsic property of a conductor denoted by ρ used to measure its resistance in the equation $R = \rho L/A$, where L is the length of the conductor and A is its cross-sectional area.

Bonding

A rule stating that atoms—except a few such as Be, H, and B—tend to react in order to form a complete octet of valence electrons. Hydrogen can have a maximum of 2 valence electrons, Be can have 4 valence electrons, and B can have 6 valence electrons.

RESISTIVITY

Physics

General Chemistry

POLAR COVALENT BOND

DC and AC Circuits

The natural tendency of a conductor to block current flow to a certain extent resulting in loss of energy or potential. Resistance is equal to the ratio of the voltage applied to the resulting current.

Bonding

A type of covalent bond between atoms with different electronegativities that results in an unequal sharing of electron pairs, giving the bond partial positive and negative poles.

RESISTANCE

Physics

General Chemistry

RESONANCE STRUCTURES

DC and AC Circuits

The rate at which the energy of flowing charges through a resistor is dissipated, given by the equation $P = IV$.

Bonding

Alternate Lewis structures of the same molecule that show the delocalization of electrons within that molecule; Lewis structures that contribute to a resonance-stabilized system. Resonance structures have the same atomic connectivity but differ in the distribution of electrons.

POWER DISSIPATED BY RESISTOR

Physics

General Chemistry

VSEPR

DC and AC Circuits

A term denoted by ε_0 used in the calculation of capacitance, given by the equation $C = \varepsilon_0 A/d$, where A is the area of one plate and d is the distance between the plates.

Bonding

The acronym for Valence Shell Electron Pair Repulsion theory, which states that the three-dimensional molecular geometry about some central atom is determined by the electronic repulsions between its bonding and nonbonding electron pairs.

PERMITTIVITY OF FREE SPACE, ε_0

Physics

General Chemistry

COMBINATION REACTION

DC and AC Circuits

Law stating that the voltage drop across a resistor is proportional to the current flowing through it, given by the equation $V = I R$.

Compounds and Stoichiometry

A reaction in which two or more reactants combine to form a product. Ex: A + B → C.

OHM'S LAW

Physics

General Chemistry

DECOMPOSITION REACTION

DC and AC Circuits

A.) In accordance with the conservation of electric charge, the sum of currents directed into a node or junction point in a circuit equals the sum of the currents directed away from that point.

B.) The sum of the voltage sources in a circuit loop is equal to the sum of voltage drops along that loop.

Compounds and Stoichiometry

A chemical reaction in which one substance breaks down into two substances.
Ex: $C \rightarrow A + B$.

KIRCHHOFF'S LAWS

Physics

DISPROPORTIONATION

A material in which electrons cannot move freely.

Compounds and Stoichiometry

A Redox reaction in which the same species is both oxidized and reduced.

INSULATOR

Physics

DOUBLE DISPLACEMENT REACTION

The voltage created by a potential difference between the two terminals of a cell when no current is flowing.

Compounds and Stoichiometry

A chemical reaction in which two different compounds exchange an atom or ion to form two new compounds; a.k.a. metathesis reaction. Ex: AB + CD → AC + BD.

ELECTRON VOLT

Physics

General Chemistry

EMPIRICAL FORMULA

DC and AC Circuits

The energy gained by an electron when it is accelerated through a potential difference of 1 Volt, given by qV where q is 1.6×10^{-19} C and V is 1 Volt.

Compounds and Stoichiometry

Chemical formula showing the smallest whole-number ratio of atoms in a compound.

ELECTROMOTIVE FORCE

Physics

General Chemistry

FORMULA WEIGHT

DC and AC Circuits

A conducting pathway that contains one or more voltage sources that drive an electric current along that pathway and through connected passive circuit elements (such as resistors).

Compounds and Stoichiometry

The sum of all the masses (in amu) present in one molecule of a molecular compound.

ELECTRIC CIRCUIT

Physics

General Chemistry

LIMITING REAGENT

DC and AC Circuits

Current that flows through a conductor in one direction only.

Compounds and Stoichiometry

The reactant of a chemical equation that, given nonstoichiometric amounts, determines the amount of product that can form; the reactant that runs out first.

DIRECT CURRENT

Physics

General Chemistry

MOLECULAR FORMULA

DC and AC Circuits

A dimensionless number that indicates the factor by which capacitance is increased when a dielectric is placed in between the plates of a capacitor, given by: $C' = KC$, where C' is the new capacitance.

Compounds and Stoichiometry

A chemical formula showing the actual number of atoms present in a certain compound.

DIELECTRIC CONSTANT

Physics

General Chemistry

MOLECULE

DC and AC Circuits

An insulating material placed in between the two plates of a capacitor. If the circuit is plugged into a current source, more charge will be stored in the capacitor. If the circuit is not plugged into a current source, the voltage of the capacitor will decrease.

Compounds and Stoichiometry

The smallest unit of a substance, composed of two or more atoms joined in covalent bonds, which still retains all the chemical properties of that substance.

DIELECTRIC

Physics

General Chemistry

NET IONIC EQUATION

DC and AC Circuits

A material in which electrons can move with relative ease.

Compounds and Stoichiometry

A representation of a displacement reaction showing only the reactive species and omitting the spectator ions.

CONDUCTOR

Physics

General Chemistry

PERCENT COMPOSITION

DC and AC Circuits

An electric device used in circuits that is basically composed of two conducting plates separated by a short distance and works to store electric charge.

Compounds and Stoichiometry

The percentages by mass (in amu) of the elements making up a compound.

CAPACITOR

Physics

General Chemistry

PERCENT YIELD

DC and AC Circuits

A measure (expressed in SI units of Farads) of a capacitor's ability to store charge, calculated by the ratio of the magnitude of charge on one plate to the voltage across the two plates.

Compounds and Stoichiometry

A ratio (calculated as a percentage) of the actual mass of product yielded to the theoretical yield of product mass.

CAPACITANCE

Physics

General Chemistry

SINGLE DISPLACEMENT REACTION

DC and AC Circuits

Current that flows through a conductor in two directions that are periodically altered.

Compounds and Stoichiometry

A chemical reaction in which an atom or ion of one compound is replaced by another atom or ion. Ex: $A + BC \rightarrow B + AC$.

ALTERNATING CURRENT

Physics

General Chemistry

THEORETICAL YIELD

Magnetism

The magnetic field produced at a perpendicular distance r from a straight current-carrying wire, calculated by the equation: $B = \mu_0 i / 2\pi r$

Compounds and Stoichiometry

The expected amount of product yielded in a reaction according to reactants' stoichiometry.

STRAIGHT-WIRE MAGNETIC FIELD

Physics

ACTIVATION ENERGY

Magnetism

A common method used to determine the direction of the magnetic force vector. The thumb points in the direction of the charge's velocity, the fingers point in the direction on the magnetic (B) field, and the palm points in the direction of the acting force.

Kinetics and Equilibrium

Often denoted by E_a, it is the energy barrier that must be overcome for a reaction to proceed.

RIGHT-HAND RULE

Physics

Magnetism

Term denoted by μ_0 and equal to $4\pi \times 10^{-7}$ Tesla meter/Ampere; used in the equation measuring the magnetic field produced by a current-carrying wire, $B = \mu_0 I/2\pi r$.

CHEMICAL KINETICS

Kinetics and Equilibrium

The study of reaction rates and the factors that affect them.

PERMEABILITY OF FREE SPACE, μ_0

Physics

COLLISION THEORY OF CHEMICAL KINETICS

Magnetism

A material whose atoms have a net magnetic field and, under conditions that allow the alignment of the individual magnetic fields, exhibits an attraction toward the pole of a magnet.

Kinetics and Equilibrium

Theory stating that the rate of a reaction is directly proportional to the number of collisions that take place between reactants per second.

PARAMAGNETIC MATERIAL

Physics

Magnetism

Equation used to measure the force exerted on a current-carrying wire due to a magnetic field, given by $F = I\,L\,B\sin\theta$, where I is the current, L is the length of the wire, B is the magnitude of the magnetic field, and θ is the angle at which the wire intersect the B-field vectors.

Kinetics and Equilibrium

A dynamic point reached by a reversible reaction in which the rate of the forward reaction is equal to the rate of the reverse reaction. There is no net change in the concentrations of the products and reactants being formed.

MAGNETIC FORCE ON CURRENT-CARRYING WIRE

Physics

EQUILIBRIUM CONSTANT

Magnetism

A force exerted on a charged particle moving through a magnetic field, calculated using the equation $F_B = q\ v\ B\ \sin\theta$, where the angle denotes that only charges moving perpendicular to the magnetic field experience a force.

Kinetics and Equilibrium

A ratio of the concentrations of the products to the concentrations of the reactants at the point of equilibrium, where each reactant and product in the expression is raised to the power of its stoichiometric coefficient. Commonly denoted by K_{eq}.

MAGNETIC FORCE

Physics

LE CHATELIER'S PRINCIPLE

Magnetism

Field vectors created by moving charges and permanent magnets that in turn exert a magnetic force on moving charges and current carrying wires.

Kinetics and Equilibrium

The fact that when a system in equilibrium is placed under one of several stressors, it will react in order to regain equilibrium.

MAGNETIC FIELD

Physics

General Chemistry

RATE-DETERMINING STEP

Magnetism

The magnetic field produced at the center of a circular loop of current-carrying wire with a radius of r, calculated by the equation: $B = \mu_0 i / 2r$.

Kinetics and Equilibrium

The slowest step in a reaction mechanism that determines the overall rate of the reaction.

LOOP-WIRE MAGNETIC FIELD

Physics

General Chemistry

RATE LAW

Magnetism

A material whose atoms have net magnetic field and, below a critical temperature, are strongly attracted to a magnet pole.

Kinetics and Equilibrium

An experimentally determined mathematical expression showing the rate of a reaction as a function of the concentration of its reactants.

Physics

FERROMAGNETIC

General Chemistry

REACTION MECHANISM

Magnetism

A material whose atoms have no net magnetic field and is therefore repelled from the pole of a magnet.

Kinetics and Equilibrium

A "play-by-play" showing the individual steps of a reaction, including the formation and destruction of any reaction intermediates that may occur.

Physics

DIAMAGNETIC MATERIAL

General Chemistry

REACTION ORDER

Magnetism

The flow of charge as it moves across a potential difference (voltage), denoted *I* and measured by the amount of charge passing through a conductor over a unit of time: $\Delta q/\Delta t$.

Kinetics and Equilibrium

The sum of the exponents in a rate law, where each exponent provides the reaction order with respect to its reactant.

CURRENT

Physics

General Chemistry

REACTION QUOTIENT

Electrostatics

The difference in electric potential between two points in an electric field, also termed the voltage (ΔV).

Kinetics and Equilibrium

A ratio of the concentrations of the products to the concentrations of the reactants at any point during the reaction aside from equilibrium, where each reactant and product in the expression is raised to the power of it stoichiometric coefficient. Commonly denoted by Q.

POTENTIAL DIFFERENCE

Physics

REACTION RATE

Electrostatics

The smallest measured electric charge, belonging to an electron; -1.6×10^{-19} C.

Kinetics and Equilibrium

The measure of how quickly reactants are consumed and products are formed, commonly expressed in terms of mol L^{-1} s^{-1}.

FUNDAMENTAL UNIT OF CHARGE

Physics

General Chemistry

REVERSIBLE REACTION

Electrostatics

Concentric circles emanating from a source charge that cross its electric field lines perpendicularly. No work is required for a test charge to travel along the circumference of an equipotential line since the potential at every point along that line is the same.

Kinetics and Equilibrium

A process that will proceed bidirectionally to form both product and reactant.

EQUIPOTENTIAL LINES

Physics

Electrostatics

The study of electric charges at rest or in motion and the forces between them.

TRANSITION STATE

General Chemistry

Kinetics and Equilibrium

A high energy complex in which old bonds are partially broken and new bonds are partially formed. Charges existing only prior to or after the formation of the complex are designated as partial charges.

ELECTROSTATICS

Physics

General Chemistry

ADIABATIC PROCESS

Electrostatics

The amount of work required to bring a test charge q_0 from infinity to a point within the electric field of some source charge Q, given by the equation $EPE = q_0V$.

Thermochemistry

A process that occurs in which no heat is transferred to or from the system by its surroundings.

ELECTRIC POTENTIAL ENERGY

Physics

General Chemistry

CLOSED SYSTEM

Electrostatics

The amount of electric potential energy per unit charge; the work required to bring a positive test charge q_0 from infinity to within an electric field of another positive source charge, Q, divided by that test charge, calculated by the equation $V = kQ / r$.

Thermochemistry

A system that allows for the exchange of energy but not matter across its boundaries.

ELECTRIC POTENTIAL

Physics

General Chemistry

CONSTANT-VOLUME CALORIMETER

Electrostatics

Imaginary lines that show the direction in which a positive test charge is accelerated by the coulombic force due to the electric field of a source charge.

Thermochemistry

An apparatus commonly referred to as a "bomb calorimeter" used to measure the amount of heat absorbed or released following a reaction.

ELECTRIC FIELD LINES

Physics

General Chemistry

ENDOTHERMIC REACTION

Electrostatics

The electrostatic force that a source charge q_s would exert on a positive test charge q_0 within its proximity divided by that test charge; $E = F_{coul} / q_0$.

Thermochemistry

A reaction that proceeds with the net absorption of energy (heat) from the surroundings.

ELECTRIC FIELD

Physics

General Chemistry

ENTHALPY

Electrostatics

The result of having two charges of opposite sign and equal magnitude separated by a short distance d.

Thermochemistry

The total heat content of a system at a constant pressure, commonly denoted by "H."

ELECTRIC DIPOLE

Physics

General Chemistry

ENTROPY

Electrostatics

A vector quantity resulting from an electric dipole, equal to the product of the charge magnitude q and the distance separating the two charges d, often denoted by p.

Thermochemistry

The chaos or randomness of a system, often denoted by the letter "S." ΔS represents the change in entropy following a reaction.

DIPOLE MOMENT

Physics

General Chemistry

EXOTHERMIC

Electrostatics

The law describing the electrostatic force that exists between two charges, q_1 and q_2, given by the equation $F_{coul} = kq_1q_2 / r^2$.

Thermochemistry

A reaction that proceeds with the net release of energy (heat) into the surroundings.

COULOMB'S LAW

Physics

General Chemistry

GIBBS FREE ENERGY

Electrostatics

The SI unit of electric charge, denoted by C.

Thermochemistry

The energy of a system available to do work.

COULOMB

Physics

General Chemistry

GIBBS-HELMHOLTZ EQUATION

Fluids and Solids

A term used in characterizing the elasticity of a solid, denoted by Y and measured by the ratio of the stress (F/A) to strain ($\Delta L/L$). Results when force is applied perpendicular to the surface area.

Thermochemistry

$$\Delta G = \Delta H - T\Delta S$$

YOUNG'S MODULUS

Physics

HEAT

Fluids and Solids

The measure of internal friction in a fluid, often denoted by η.

Thermochemistry

A transferable energy usually in the form of kinetic energy of molecules.

VISCOSITY

Physics

General Chemistry

HESS'S LAW

Fluids and Solids

Type of liquid flow that occurs when the flow rate in a tube exceeds V_c. The motion of the fluid that is not adjacent to the container walls is highly irregular, forming vortices and a high flow resistance.

Thermochemistry

A statement that the enthalpy change of an overall reaction is equal to the sum of the standard heats of formation of the products minus the sum of the standard heats of formation of the reactants.

TURBULENT FLOW

Physics

ISOBARIC PROCESS

Lines that trace out the path of a water particles as they flow in a tube without ever crossing each other.

Thermochemistry

A process that occurs at a constant pressure.

STREAMLINE

Physics

General Chemistry

ISOCHORIC PROCESS

Fluids and Solids

A dimensionless quantity given by the density of a substance divided by the density of water, where ρ_{water} = 1 g/mL or 1 g/cm^3.

Thermochemistry

A process in which volume remains constant and no net pressure-volume work is done.

SPECIFIC GRAVITY

Physics

General Chemistry

ISOLATED SYSTEM

Fluids and Solids

A term describing a solid's resistance to shear stress, denoted by S and measured by the ratio of shear stress (F/A) to strain (x/h). Results when a force is applied parallel to the surface area.

Thermochemistry

A system that can exchange neither energy nor matter with its surroundings.

SHEAR MODULUS

Physics

General Chemistry

ISOTHERMAL PROCESS

Fluids and Solids

Principle stating that when a pressure is applied to one point of an enclosed fluid, that pressure is transmitted in equal magnitude to all points within that fluid and to the walls of its container. This principle forms the basis of the hydraulic lift.

Thermochemistry

A process that occurs in which the system either gains or loses energy in order to maintain a constant temperature.

PASCAL'S PRINCIPLE

Physics

LAW OF CONSERVATION OF ENERGY

Fluids and Solids

The simplest type of liquid flow through a tube where thin layers of liquid slide over one another, occurring as long as the flow rate remains below a critical velocity V_C.

Thermochemistry

Law stating that energy cannot be created nor destroyed but only transferred and transformed.

LAMINAR FLOW

Physics

General Chemistry

OPEN SYSTEM

Fluids and Solids

The pressure above the atmospheric pressure, given only by $\rho g z$; the difference between $P_{absolute}$ and P_0.

Thermochemistry

A system that allows for the exchange of energy and matter across its boundaries.

GAUGE PRESSURE

Physics

General Chemistry

SPECIFIC HEAT

Fluids and Solids

A scalar quantity defined as the mass per unit volume, often denoted by ρ.

Thermochemistry

The amount of heat required to raise one gram of a substance by 1 degree Celsius; heat capacity.

DENSITY

Physics

General Chemistry

SPONTANEOUS REACTION

Fluids and Solids

The equation following the law that the mass flow rate of fluid must remain constant from one cross-section of a tube to another, given by $A_1V_1 = A_2V_2$.

Thermochemistry

A reaction that will proceed or occur on its own without an input of energy from its surroundings.

CONTINUITY EQUATION

Physics

General Chemistry

STANDARD FREE ENERGY

Fluids and Solids

A type of attractive force felt by liquid molecules toward each other. Cohesion is responsible for surface tension.

Thermochemistry

The value of ΔG as calculated under standard conditions: at 1 atmosphere (atm) and 0 Kelvin.

COHESION

Physics

General Chemistry

STANDARD HEAT OF FORMATION

Fluids and Solids

A term that describes a fluid's resistance to compression under a pressure, denoted by B and measured by the ratio of stress (pressure change) to strain; ΔP / $(\Delta V/V)$.

Thermochemistry

Measure of the heat absorbed or released when a substance is formed from its naturally occurring elements. Often denoted by ΔH_f.

BULK MODULUS

Physics

General Chemistry

STANDARD HEAT OF REACTION

Fluids and Solids

Equation describing the conservation of energy in fluid flow, given by

$P_1 + 1/2\ \rho V_1^2 + \rho g y_1 = P_2 + 1/2\ \rho v_2^2 + \rho g y_2$.

Thermochemistry

The change in enthalpy of a reaction at STP.

BERNOULLI'S EQUATION

Physics

General Chemistry

STATE FUNCTION

Fluids and Solids

A body that is fully or partially immersed in a liquid will be buoyed up by a force that is equal to the weight of the liquid displaced by the body. $F_{buoyant} = \rho_{liq}\, g\, V_{liq} = \rho_{obj}\, g\, V_{obj}$, where V_{obj} is the volume of the object submerged.

Thermochemistry

A function that depends only on the initial and final states of a system, not on the path in between.

Physics

ARCHIMEDES' PRINCIPLE

General Chemistry

SYSTEM

Fluids and Solids

A type of attractive force that molecules of a liquid feel toward molecules of another substance, such as in the adhesion of water droplets to a glass surface.

Thermochemistry

The part of the universe under consideration that is separated by some real or imaginary boundary from its surroundings.

ADHESION

Physics

General Chemistry

AVOGADRO'S PRINCIPLE

Fluids and Solids

The pressure below the surface of a liquid that depends on gravity and surface pressure, calculated by $P = P_0 + \rho g z$, where P is the absolute pressure, z is depth, and P_0 is the surface pressure.

The Gas Phase

Principle stating that when different gases of equal volumes are at identical temperatures and pressures, they contain equal numbers of molecules.

ABSOLUTE PRESSURE

BOYLE'S LAW

Thermodynamics

The expansion in volume of a liquid as a result of increasing temperatures, calculated by the equation $\Delta V = \beta V \Delta T$, where V is volume and β is the coefficient of volume expansion.

The Gas Phase

At a constant temperature, the volume of an ideal gas is inversely proportional to its pressure. $V \propto 1/P$.

VOLUME EXPANSION

Physics

CHARLES AND GAY-LUSSAC LAW

Thermodynamics

The study of heat transfer and its effects.

The Gas Phase

At a constant pressure, the volume of an ideal gas is directly proportional to its temperature. $V \alpha T$.

THERMODYNAMICS

Physics

General Chemistry

DIFFUSION

Thermodynamics

The expansion of a solid as a result of increasing temperatures, calculated by the equation $\Delta L = \alpha L \Delta T$, where L is the length, α is the coefficient of linear expansion, and T is the temperature.

The Gas Phase

Passive transport of a gas or solute throughout a medium by means of random motion.

THERMAL EXPANSION

Physics

General Chemistry

EFFUSION

Thermodynamics

A measure of the heat content that a body possesses measured on either the Kelvin, Celsius, or Fahrenheit scale.

The Gas Phase

The movement of gas through a small opening into an area of lower pressure.

TEMPERATURE

Physics

General Chemistry

GRAHAM'S LAW

Thermodynamics

When a thermodynamic process moves a system from one state of equilibrium to another, the entropy (S) of that system combined with that of its surroundings will either increase or remain unchanged; for irreversible processes entropy will increase and for reversible processes entropy will not change.

The Gas Phase

Law stating that the rate at which two different gases effuse/diffuse is inversely proportional to the square-root of their molecular weight. $R_1/R_2 = (MM_2/MM_1)^{1/2}$.

SECOND LAW OF THERMODYNAMICS

Physics

General Chemistry

HENRY'S LAW

Thermodynamics

Form of heat transfer accomplished by electromagnetic waves, which can travel through a vacuum.

The Gas Phase

The partial pressure of a gas dissolved in a solution is directly proportional to the partial pressure of this gas above the solution.

Physics

RADIATION

General Chemistry

IDEAL GAS

Thermodynamics

The force per unit area: F/A.

The Gas Phase

A hypothetical gas whose particles would occupy zero volume and have no attractive intermolecular forces.

PRESSURE

Physics

General Chemistry

IDEAL GAS LAW

Thermodynamics

The most commonly used temperature scale (SI units) that ranges up from absolute zero.

$T_K = T_C + 273.$

The Gas Phase

A unification of Boyle's Law, Charles' Law, and Avogadro's Principle into the formula that describes the behavior of ideal gases: PV = nRT.

KELVIN

Physics

General Chemistry

KINETIC MOLECULAR THEORY OF GASES

Thermodynamics

The heat of transformation corresponding to a phase change from liquid to gas or from gas to liquid.

The Gas Phase

A series of ideas used to account for the behavior of ideal gases. The theory describes gas as volumeless particles in constant, random motion that exhibit no intermolecular attractions and undergo completely elastic collisions with each other and their container walls.

HEAT OF VAPORIZATION

Physics

Thermodynamics

The amount of heat required to change the phase of a substance, calculated by the equation $q = mL$, where q is heat, m is the mass of the substance, and L is the heat of transformation for that substance.

PARTIAL PRESSURE

General Chemistry

The Gas Phase

The pressure contribution of single gas in a container holding a mixture of gases, as given by the equation $P_A = P_{total}X_A$, where X_A is the mole fraction of gas "A" and P_{total} is the total pressure of the mixture.

HEAT OF TRANSFORMATION

Physics

STP

Thermodynamics

The heat of transformation corresponding to a phase change from either solid to liquid or from liquid to solid.

The Gas Phase

273 Kelvin (0° Celsius) and 1 atmosphere (760 torr).

HEAT OF FUSION

Physics

General Chemistry

VAPOR PRESSURE

Thermodynamics

The change in internal energy of a system (ΔU) is equal to the heat (Q) transferred into the system minus the energy lost by the system when it performs work (W). $\Delta U = Q - W$.

The Gas Phase

The partial pressure of a vapor when it is in equilibrium with its solid or liquid phase.

FIRST LAW OF THERMODYNAMICS

Physics

General Chemistry

AZEOTROPE

Thermodynamics

Form of heat transfer applying only to fluids (liquids and gases) where heated material transfers energy by bulk flow and physical motion.

Phase and Phase Changes

A liquid mixture of two or more substances that has a constant boiling point greater than or less than the boiling points of its constituents. The vapor of this unique mixture has the same composition as the liquid state making it difficult to separate the constituents.

CONVECTION

Physics

General Chemistry

COLLIGATIVE PROPERTIES

Thermodynamics

Form of heat transfer where heat energy is directly transferred between molecules through molecular collisions or direct contact.

Phase and Phase Changes

The properties of solutions—such as vapor pressure lowering, freezing point depression, boiling point elevation, and osmotic pressure—that are affected only by the number of solute particles dissolved and not their chemical identities.

CONDUCTION

Physics

General Chemistry

PHASE DIAGRAM

Thermodynamics

A unit of heat (C) that equals 10^3 calories (c) or 4,184 Joules.

Phase and Phase Changes

A pressure versus temperature plot showing the conditions under which a substance exists in equilibrium between different phases or in which the substance exists in pure phase.

CALORIE

Physics

General Chemistry

RAOULT'S LAW

Work, Energy, and Momentum

A theorem stating that the net work performed on an object is related to the change in kinetic energy of that body, given by the equation $W = \Delta KE$.

Phase and Phase Changes

The vapor pressure of one component above a solution is proportional to the mole fraction of that component in the solution. $P_A = X_A P_{total}$.

WORK-ENERGY THEOREM

Physics

General Chemistry

TRIPLE POINT

Work, Energy, and Momentum

The quantity measured when a constant force acts on a body to move it a distance d, calculated by the equation Work = F d $\cos\theta$, where $\cos\theta$ indicates that only the component of the force parallel to the direction of motion is considered.

Phase and Phase Changes

A point on a phase diagram at which a substance exists in equilibrium between all three phases.

WORK

Physics

General Chemistry

AQUEOUS SOLUTION

Work, Energy, and Momentum

The rate at which work is done, given by the equation Power = $W/\Delta t$, where W is work and t is time (in seconds).

Solutions

A solution containing water as its solvent.

POWER

Physics

General Chemistry

COMMON ION EFFECT

Work, Energy, and Momentum

The energy of an object due to its height off ground level, calculated by the equation PE = mgh.

Solutions

The molar solubility of one salt is reduced when another salt, having a common ion, is brought into the same solution.

POTENTIAL ENERGY

Physics

General Chemistry

CONCENTRATION

Work, Energy, and Momentum

A force, such as friction, which performs work over a distance that is dependent on the path taken between the initial and final positions.

Solutions

A ratio of the amount of solute to the amount of solution.

NONCONSERVATIVE FORCE

Physics

General Chemistry

ELECTROLYTE

Work, Energy, and Momentum

Often denoted by p, it is a vector quantity given by an object's mass times its velocity.

Solutions

A compound ionizing in water that is capable of conducting electricity in that solution.

Physics

MOMENTUM

Work, Energy, and Momentum

The energy of an object in motion, calculated by the equation $KE = 1/2\ mv^2$ and given in the SI unit of Joules (J).

ION

General Chemistry

Solutions

A single or polyatomic particle with an electric charge.

KINETIC ENERGY

Physics

ION PRODUCT

Often denoted by J, it is the change in momentum, given by Δp.

Solutions

The product of the molar concentrations of dissociated ions in solution at any point in the reaction other than equilibrium or saturation, where each ion is raised to the power of its stoichiometric coefficient. Denoted “IP.”

IMPULSE

Physics

General Chemistry

MOLALITY

Work, Energy, and Momentum

A force, such as gravity, which performs work over a distance that is independent of the path taken.

Solutions

Concentration of a solution calculated by (mole solute)/(1kg solvent).

CONSERVATIVE FORCE

Physics

General Chemistry

MOLARITY

Work, Energy, and Momentum

The momentum of a system remains constant when there are no net external forces acting on it.

Solutions

Concentration of a solution calculated by (mole solute)/(L solution).

CONSERVATION OF MOMENTUM

Physics

MOLAR SOLUBILITY

Work, Energy, and Momentum

When only conservative forces act on an object and work is done, energy is conserved and described by the equation: $\Delta E = \Delta KE + \Delta PE = 0$.

Solutions

The molar amount of a solute that can dissolve in 1 L of solvent until equilibrium—saturation—is reached.

CONSERVATION OF MECHANICAL ENERGY

Physics

General Chemistry

NORMALITY

Work, Energy, and Momentum

Type of collision in which the two bodies stick together after colliding, resulting in one final mass and velocity. Momentum is conserved but kinetic energy is not.

Solutions

The gram equivalent weight of solute per liter of solution, often denoted by N.

COMPLETELY INELASTIC COLLISIONS

Physics

General Chemistry

SOLUBILITY

Work, Energy, and Momentum

Type of collision in which both momentum and kinetic energy are conserved. That is, the sum of the initial kinetic energies right before the collision equals the sum of the final kinetic energies just after the collision.

Solutions

A ratio that measures how much solute can dissolve in a solvent at a given temperature, expressed in units of (g solute)/(100 g solvent).

COMPLETELY ELASTIC COLLISIONS

Physics

SOLUBILITY PRODUCT CONSTANT

Work, Energy, and Momentum

The point on some object or body at which all of its mass is considered to be concentrated.

Solutions

The product of the molar concentrations of dissociated ions in solution at saturation, where each ion is raised to the power of its stoichiometric coefficient. Denoted K_{sp}.

CENTER OF MASS

Physics

General Chemistry

SOLUTE

Work, Energy, and Momentum

The point on some object or body at which the entire force of gravity is considered to act on.

Solutions

A compound, commonly a solid, dissolved in a solvent to create a solution.

CENTER OF GRAVITY

Physics

SOLUTION EQUILIBRIUM

Newtonian Mechanics

A force that measures the gravitational pull on an object, given by the object's mass times its gravitational acceleration; mg, where g is 9.8 m/s^2 as measured on Earth.

Solutions

When a solute is dissolved in a solvent it will dissociate until reaching an equilibrium point at which the rate of dissociation equals the rate of precipitation of the solute, regardless of any additional solute introduced into the mixture.

WEIGHT

Physics

General Chemistry

SOLVATION

Newtonian Mechanics

State where the sum of the forces acting on an object is zero, giving it no net acceleration.

Solutions

A cagelike network of solvent molecules that forms around a solute in a solution.

TRANSLATIONAL EQUILIBRIUM

Physics

General Chemistry

SOLVENT

Newtonian Mechanics

The magnitude of a force acting on a body times the perpendicular distance between the acting force and the axis of rotation, denoted by τ with the SI units N m.

Solutions

A medium, commonly a liquid, into which a solute is dissolved to create a solution.

TORQUE

Physics

General Chemistry

ACID DISSOCIATION CONSTANT

Newtonian Mechanics

State where the sum of the torques acting on a body is zero, giving it no net angular acceleration.

Acids and Bases

An equilibrium expression used to measure weak-acid strength, given by the ratio of the product of the products' molar concentrations to the product of the reactants' molar concentrations, with each term raised to the power of its stoichiometric coefficient. Denoted K_a.

ROTATIONAL EQUILIBRIUM

Physics

General Chemistry

AMPHOTERIC

Newtonian Mechanics

Perpendicular component of the force caused when two surfaces push against each other, denoted by F_N.

Acids and Bases

A species capable of reacting with either an H^+ or OH^-, thereby behaving as either an acid or a base; amphiprotic.

NORMAL FORCE

Physics

General Chemistry

ARRHENIUS DEFINITION

Newtonian Mechanics

If body A exerts a force F_A on body B, then body B exerts a force that is equal in magnitude but opposite in direction to F_A, called $-F_A$; the law of "action and reaction."

Acids and Bases

A definition of acids as producers of H^+ and bases as producers of OH^- in aqueous solution.

NEWTON'S THIRD LAW

Physics

BRONSTED-LOWRY DEFINITION

Newtonian Mechanics

When a net force acts on a body it will have a net acceleration pointing in the direction of the net force that is proportional to the body's mass in the following relationship: $F_{net} = ma_{net}$.

Acids and Bases

Common definition of acids as proton (H^+) donors and bases as proton acceptors.

NEWTON'S SECOND LAW

Physics

General Chemistry

BUFFER

Newtonian Mechanics

If a body has either a zero or constant speed, it will remain that way unless a net force acts upon it.

Acids and Bases

A solution containing a weak acid or base coupled with its conjugate salt, acting to prevent changes to the solution's pH upon the addition of acidic or basic substances.

NEWTON'S FIRST LAW

Physics

General Chemistry

CONJUGATE ACIDS AND BASES

Newtonian Mechanics

A scalar quantity used as a measure of an object's inertia.

Acids and Bases

A systematic pairing of a deprotonated specie (base) with its protonated form (conjugate acid). Conjugates appear on opposite sides of a chemical equation.

MASS

Physics

General Chemistry

DIPROTIC BASE

Newtonian Mechanics

A ubiquitous attractive force existing between any two objects, whose magnitude is directly proportional to the product of the two masses observed and inversely proportional to the square of their distance.

Acids and Bases

A base that can accept two moles of H^+ per mole of itself. Ex: SO_4^{2-}.

GRAVITY

Physics

General Chemistry

EQUIVALENCE POINT

Newtonian Mechanics

An antagonistic force that points parallel and opposite in direction to the movement (or attempted movement) of an object.

Acids and Bases

The point in a titration at which an equimolar amount of titrant has been added to the unknown solution.

FRICTION FORCE

Physics

General Chemistry

HALF-EQUIVALENCE POINT

Newtonian Mechanics

A vector quantity describing the push or pull on an object. The SI unit for force is the Newton (N).

Acids and Bases

The point in a titration at which exactly half the molar equivalence of reactant is consumed by the titrant being added. At this point in an acid-base titration, the pK of the unknown solution is revealed. pK = pH of the solution at half-equivalence point during the titration.

FORCE

Physics

General Chemistry

HENDERSON-HASSELBACH EQUATION

Newtonian Mechanics

The acceleration of an object traveling in a circle with a constant speed, equal in magnitude to the velocity squared divided by the radius of the circle traversed. The direction of the acceleration always points toward the center of the circle.

Acids and Bases

An equation commonly used in titration-based problems that relates the pH or pOH of a solution to the pK and the ratio of the dissociated species. $pH = pKa + \log ([A^{-}]/–[HA])$.

CENTRIPETAL ACCELERATION

Physics

Units and Kinematics

A vector quantity describing an object's displacement over the elapsed time, written:
$v = \Delta x/\Delta t$.

INDICATOR

General Chemistry

Acids and Bases

A chemical species that changes color when undergoing disassociation. Indicators are used to signal the end point of a titration.

VELOCITY

Physics

General Chemistry

LEWIS DEFINITION

Units and Kinematics

A quantity that has both magnitude and direction.

Acids and Bases

A definition of acids as electron-pair acceptors and bases as electron-pair donors.

General Chemistry

NEUTRALIZATION REACTION

Units and Kinematics

A scalar quantity describing the distance traveled over the time required to travel that distance.

Acids and Bases

A reaction in which an acid and a base are combined to form water and a salt.

SPEED

Physics

General Chemistry

pH

Units and Kinematics

A quantity that only has a magnitude but no direction.

Acids and Bases

Scaled value used to measure the acidic strength of a solution, calculated by taking the negative logarithm (–log) of the H^+ molar concentration of a solution. $pH = -\log [H^+]$

SCALAR

Physics

Units and Kinematics

A vector quantity describing the straight-line distance between an initial and final position of some particle or object.

General Chemistry

pl

Acids and Bases

The pH of a molecule at which it contains no net electric charge; isoelectric point.

DISPLACEMENT

Physics

General Chemistry

STRONG ACIDS

Units and Kinematics

A vector quantity describing a change in velocity over the elapsed time for which that change occurs, written: $a = \Delta v / \Delta t$.

Acids and Bases

An acid that will completely dissociate in aqueous solution. Ex: HCl; HI; $HClO_4$.

ACCELERATION

Physics

General Chemistry

TITRATION

Redox Reactions and Electrochemistry

The tendency of a species to be reduced, as measured at 25°C when reacting species are of 1M concentration or 1atm partial pressure (for gases).

Acids and Bases

An analytical procedure in which a solution of known concentration is slowly added to a solution of unknown concentration to the point of molar equivalency, thereby providing the concentration of the unknown solution.

STANDARD REDUCTION POTENTIAL

General Chemistry

General Chemistry

WATER DISSOCIATION CONSTANT

Redox Reactions and Electrochemistry

The difference between the two reduction potentials of half-cells in a cell under standard conditions, i.e., 25°C; 1M and 1atm concentrations. Given by: $E^{o}_{cell} = E^{o}_{cathode} - E^{o}_{anode}$.

Acids and Bases

An expression of the auto-ionization of water into H^+ and OH^- at a certain temperature, given by the product of the ions' molar concentrations. Denoted by K_w, and equal to 10^{-14} at 25°C. $K_w = [H^+] [OH^-]$

STANDARD ELECTROMOTIVE FORCE

General Chemistry

General Chemistry

ANODE

Redox Reactions and Electrochemistry

A measure of the tendency of a species to be reduced, commonly used in identifying the anode and cathode of an electrochemical cell.

Redox Reactions and Electrochemistry

The electrode at which oxidation occurs during a cell's redox reaction. Electrons always flow from the anode in an electrochemical cell.

REDUCTION POTENTIAL

General Chemistry

General Chemistry

CATHODE

A reaction in which a species gains electrons.

Redox Reactions and Electrochemistry

Redox Reactions and Electrochemistry

The electrode at which reduction occurs during a cell's redox reaction. Electrons always flow to the cathode in an electrochemical cell.

REDUCTION

General Chemistry

General Chemistry

ELECTROCHEMICAL REACTION

Redox Reactions and Electrochemistry

A species that is oxidized in the process of reducing another species.

Redox Reactions and Electrochemistry

A chemical reaction that is either driven by or that produces electricity.

REDUCING AGENT

General Chemistry

ELECTROLYTIC CELL

Redox Reactions and Electrochemistry

The hypothetical equation showing only the species that is oxidized or reduced in a redox reaction and the correct number of electrons transferred between the species in the complete, balanced equation.

An electrochemical cell that uses an external electric source to drive a nonspontaneous (unfavorable) redox reaction to proceed.

REDOX HALF-REACTION

General Chemistry

FARADAY'S CONSTANT

Redox Reactions and Electrochemistry

A species that is reduced in the process of oxidizing another species.

Redox Reactions and Electrochemistry

Denoted by F, it equals 9.65×10^4 coulombs/mol e^-. Commonly used in the formula: $It = n\text{F}$, where I is current, t is time (in seconds), and n is mol e^-.

OXIDIZING AGENT

General Chemistry

General Chemistry

GALVANIC CELL

Redox Reactions and Electrochemistry

A reaction in which a species loses electrons.

An electrochemical cell powered by a spontaneous redox reaction that produces an electric current flow; voltaic cell.

OXIDATION

General Chemistry

HALF-CELL

An equation used to determine a cell's electromotive force when conditions are not standard. $E_{cell} = E°_{cell} - (.0592/n) \log Q$, where n is the number of moles of electrons transferred in the redox reaction.

Redox Reactions and Electrochemistry

An electrode immersed in an electrolytic solution that is the site of either oxidation or reduction in a galvanic (voltaic) cell.

NERNST EQUATION

How Did We Do? Please Grade This Book.

Thank you for choosing a Kaplan book. Your comments and suggestions are very useful to us. Please help us in our continued development of high-quality resources to meet your needs and complete our online survey form.

www.kaplansurveys.com/books

Thank you!

KAPLAN

Test Prep and Admissions

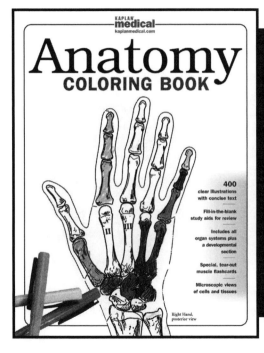

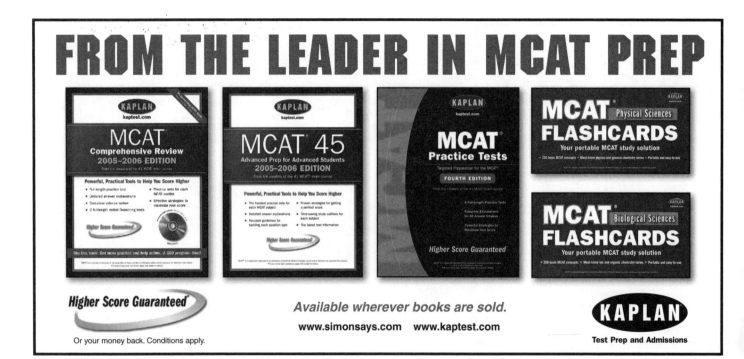